The
Attitude
Factor
In Weight loss
And Fitness

Onavire A. Ikuwan

Dedication.

Praise to God. Dedicated to all those who want to shed weight and be fit. To those who work with them and to those who create materials that will help obese and unfit people.

LEGAL NOTICE.

The author and publisher have used their best efforts in preparing this report. The author and publisher make no Representation or warranties with respect to the accuracy, applicability, fitness, or completeness of the contents of this report.

The information contained in this report is strictly for educational purposes. Therefore, if you wish to apply ideas contained

in this report, you are taking full responsibility for your actions.

Every effort has been made to accurately represent this product and it's potential.

However, there is no guarantee that you will improve in any way using the techniques

And ideas in this material.

The author and publisher disclaim any warranties (express or implied), merchantability, or fitness for any particular purpose.

The author and publisher shall in no event be held liable to any party for any direct, indirect, punitive, special, incidental or

other consequential damages arising directly or indirectly from any use of this material, which is provided "as is", and

without warranties.

As always, the advice of a competent professional should be sought.

All links (if any) are for information purposes only and are not warranted for content, accuracy or any other implied or explicit purpose.

Should there be any link, the author and publisher might earn some commission should you decide to purchase items through the link(s).

However, you are to carry out your own due diligence. The author and publisher will not be held liable for any loss, injuries and such like suffered in the course of using the products recommended.

Remember, there is no shortcut to losing weight.

1

What Is Attitude

Attitude is a common word used when referring to somebody's opinion or feeling towards something. It is somebody's personal view or general feeling of something. How the person feels towards something, and this affect their action also. Arising from this definition, you can see the power of personal action. You begin to see that your attitude can affect you a lot depending on how you align it. It could be positive or negative.

If you have a healthy opinion towards something, your body will also respond in the same line. The reverse is also the case. Here is a quote from Charles Swindoll

The longer I live, the more I realize the impact of attitude on life. Attitude, to me, is more important than facts. It is more important than the past, than education, than money, than circumstances, than failures, than successes, than what other people think or say or do. It is more important than appearance, gift or skill. It will make or break a company, a church or a home.

The remarkable thing is we have a choice every day regarding the attitude we will embrace for that day. We cannot change our past... we cannot change the fact that people will act in a certain way. We cannot change the inevitable. The only thing we can do is play on the one string we have, and that is our attitude... I am convinced that life is 10% what happens to me and 90% how I react to it. **And so it is with you... we are in charge of our attitude.**

-Charles R. Swindoll.

Let me repeat that. We are in charge of our attitude.

The Attitude Factor

The attitude factor is vital in considering the matter of weight loss and the management of it. However, some of the wisdom here can be applied to any field of human activity. Why the right attitude will get you the rights results, the wrong attitude will get you zero result.

There are all sorts of programs in this weight loss business. And obviously, different niches are targeted. Each niche will have programs of different quality. That is normal in every situation.

Most people have bought more than one program which they followed for a time and then they abandoned it. Why did they stop using the programs? Were the programs too hard or what? Whether hard or not, high quality or low, I believe the attitude of the individual towards the program and how they perceived their condition is the key reason why they did not follow through on the programs.

One thing this book wants to do is to make you aware of this and to help you to deal with it so that you can have the result you desire and deserve.

Attitude is everything

Attitude is indeed everything and on this particular matter of weight loss and fitness, it is very true. People will get things done or not, be rich or poor, be sick or healthy due mostly to their attitude. If you take a proper look at yourself, you will agree with me that your attitude has been a factor in what you have or have not achieved. If you can just have the discipline to change your attitude, you will be able to achieve much.

Changing your attitude is not done with a wave of the hand like in magic. It is worked on. Wishing will not work. You do have an experience of what I am saying here. There are certain people you have bonded well with because their actions, speech and behavior resonate well with you. There are others you have kept at arm's length or even stopped speaking to due to your disapproval of their manners. The same can be said of certain foods you choose to eat or not eat. There are places you choose to go or not. The lists go on and on. The point here is that you are used to acting in a certain way based on the circumstance. And each time your actions are conscious or unconscious.

What I seek to achieve here is to make you conscious of the actions you take in respect of weight loss and to move you to a stage where your actions become automatic and positive in respect to the subject matter. I believe it can be done. You need to believe too.

Why consider weight matters

The issue of weight loss and fitness has important implications for the overall health burden of a nation, family and individuals. Medical reports show that having excess weight and obesity are major factors that predispose one to hypertension, type 2 diabetics, sudden death, stroke , fatty liver, hypercholesterolemia, hypertriglyceridemia, arthritis, asthma, some form of cancer and other degenerative conditions. These ailments have serious economic implications for the nation, family and individuals. A hypertensive person will always be on drugs to avoid other consequences from occurring. These drugs are not cheap. Neither is it cheap to maintain diabetes which has no cure yet. Are we going to talk of stroke which totally incapacitates a person? The burden of care is also there for all those who are directly connected to the obese person. Surely, obesity and overweight are highly undesirable in any individual. It is then very important that we understand the implications of obesity and overweight and the need to deal with them. These two conditions have serious implications for national health.

2

Why are you Fat, Overweight and Unfit?

Maybe you have asked that question. Why am I fat? You will ask that

Question the more, when you know that there is negative health situations associated with being fat. So, why are you fat? Fatness does start with been overweight and the consequence is that you will be unfit. When you are unfit, you know. No one can know it like you. Overweight and obesity can start from childhood, or as somebody enters into adulthood. It can even start when one become an adult. Now, let us look at the possible reasons why you are fat.

Possible Reasons Why You are Fat

Genetic factor

Do genes play any role in fatness or obesity? The answer is not a total yes. If any of your parents or grandparents is fat or obese, there is the probability that one or more of their offspring will be fat. Having said that, it must be understood in the context of the environment. If you have the tendency to be obese and you engage in healthy life choices like eating the right food and physical exercises even of the mild type, the tendency for that obesity gene to be expressed is slim. Viewed critically in the light of current evidences, genes play a role in being fat or obese. Genes affect the amount and type of food we prefer to eat and this is where it can be tricky for those with obesity genes. The issue here then is watching your food combinations. Eat healthy. Do not starve yourself. The general report is that childhood obesity is increasing around the world and that is a time bomb because, it means type 2 diabetics will be on the rise since they are associated. And this is genetically driven. So, it is good you are reading this. Better take action now to reduce your overweight or ensure you do not become overweight.

Environment

There are regions where people are fatter than others. From recent report, 50% of the obese people in the world are from the US, China, India, Russia, Brazil, Mexico, Egypt, Germany, Pakistan and Indonesia. America Samoa, Nauru, Kuwait, Cook Islands are among the nations with highest obesity rate of 50% as at the time of putting this book together. This is surely due to the type of food that is consumed in those places. The environment provides the type of food that is available to eat. So, it does affect food choices. Some people are closer to places where processed food is sold and the tendency to go for this type of food is higher in them. You need to understand your environment to enable you make right food choices for your overall health. But my advice is that you stick to primary food sources and reduce or stop entirely all sort of processed foods and fries.

Primary foods are foods gotten direct from nature. The only process they undergo is to remove harmful chemicals, (like the process that removes cyanide from cassava. This process is purely physical), remove external coverings and such other simple processes. The conversion of grains, legumes and certain root crops to flour form is purely physical. Putting them in containers does not make them to qualify as canned foods. No chemicals are added to change the structure of the produce.

Processed foods are those that have their primary structure altered by strong heat, chemical addition, enzyme alteration and such like. In most cases, they are fried or baked. They mostly contain hydrogenated vegetable fat, high fructose corn syrup (HFCS), chemical additives, high sodium levels and high glutamate levels. When compared to natural foods, processed foods tend to be tastier, appetizing and less filling. They have more calories, more salt and primary sugars, colors and preservatives. All these make their consumption undesirable. Yet, there are people that stuff their gut with them daily.

Parental

Parents do sometimes contribute to the obese nature of their children who later grow up into adulthood in that obese condition. How? By giving their children junk food. This often happens when their financial situation changes for the better or where there is cook laziness in the home. You find that in some homes where there is a fortunate change in financial status, the kitchen is abandoned and eateries take its place. That is cook laziness. They allow the children to indulge in all sorts of foods and drinks that do not contribute to the overall health of the children. Such parents need to do an about turn and start giving their children and ward, healthy food. That way, they will have less health problems to contend with later on. If you need to combat your weight issues, you must look back at the kind of food you were eating while young, analyze them well and make changes were you need to.

For instance, what where your carbohydrate to protein ratio. What type of fats did you consume more: like saturated to unsaturated or like animal fat to plant fat. What is your attitude towards taking fruits and vegetables? What are your eating habits in between meals? Some people snack on high calorie, low quality foods like pies, doughnuts or a double meal instead of fruits. They also must take fizzy drinks everyday in place of water. You have to check back to see if you once had such eating habits and compare them with now. Note the difference and make the change for your health and fitness sake.

Peer Pressure

This should not be a surprise. Most of us know that when friends get together, most of the things they eat and drink are the things that responsible parents will not agree to. They eat more of junk food and take unhealthy drinks. They actually overindulge in such things. If they continue like that, fatness could result. I know that this is a slim factor. Now, how many people can resist peer pressure? And there is a carryover effect in peer pressure behavior. What is done by the group, majority of the individuals in the group tend to carry it out privately. Eating habit inclusive.

Personal factor

We can also be directly responsible for our condition. An individual with an undisciplined eating habit will surely end up fat and unfit. One of those habits is eating in between meals. A sort of snack factor. When you snack on pastries and fries, the result of that will be obesity. You do know of people who in their teenage years were slim but as they got more into society, they got more into junk eating and unhealthy drinks and with time, their weight ballooned and before you know it, they were fat and out of shape. They caused it and they have to take the responsibility for that.

One thing we should know in all these is that some people who are fat do see it initially as a status thing. It is when relations, friends, health professionals and fitness experts begin to point out the dangers involved that they realize how wrong they have been. When they come to this point, the battle to slim down begins. Some win it but most do not. Do you see your fatness or overweight as a problem or a status. That will determine how you deal with it. If you see it as a problem, keep reading. I will be revealing more method on how to develop the right attitude towards dealing with your weight loss and fitness problem. But if obesity is a status symbol to you. Do not bother to read further.

Depression

This can be a reason why you are fat. People talk, tease and do things that can be upsetting to you. What some people do is rather than confront the challenge, they hide behind eating. Normally, what they eat is junk food. So over time, overweight and obesity set in.

So, except you find your good point and be in control, you will lose.

3

What People Do About Their Weight and Fitness Problem

Sooner or later, most people who are fat and obese come to

realize that they have a problem. They experience constant fatigue.

There is the fast breathing that happens when small tasks are carried

out. It is like being out of breath. It is almost like what happens when a person with a healthy weight runs fast for few seconds. Entering a public vehicle is a problem. Any obese person is used to seeing the look of apprehension in the faces of passengers when they enter a public vehicle. What about the blood pressure problem. Add also the inconvenience of not eating what you like, to avoid compounding a problem. All these are some of the problems that come with being fat, overweight or obese. So, when they know that they have a problem, they begin to seek help. The first people who offer them health tips are their friends and relations. In most cases, these people do not have an expert opinion to give. They rely on what they think would work which is not supported by any research fact. When they try those prescriptions and fail to see any result, they become skeptical.

As a matter of fact, you may know some obese persons who have given up on any help. I know of some too. They just will not want to do much about their weight situation. They have perfected various excuses with which they live by and whatever you say falls on deaf ears. In the past, some of these persons relied on the prescriptions of people who did not have knowledge about weight loss reduction and management. Consequently, their prescriptions did not work and rather than seek out actual experts, some of these obese persons moved subconsciously into the realm of self pity and graduated to self justification and even defiance. So, they stopped trying, period. If you have read this far, you sure are not one of them. That is good.

Those who really want to do something about their fat or obese condition go a step further to see a doctor. He too will give his prescriptions which may or may not work. I think the reason for that is obvious. He may be a general practitioner with little interest in obesity matters. So, except he is a specialist in matters of obesity, he really may not offer much help. The difference is that, his method has the support of science. The problem here is that if his prescriptions do not worked, some patients get disillusioned and give up. And I am sure that if a study is done, the number of those who give up might be quite sizeable.

Some people enroll into gym clubs for fitness and weight loss training. Why this is good, it is not holistic and they might not get much result. The reason is because there are a whole lot of factors to be considered and going in one direction will not solve the problem. It is proven that exercise cannot really help people to lose weight though it may help them to keep fit. What exercise can a severely obese person do that will help if it is not combined with diet and even surgery. So, like I said, going in one direction will not work. Flowing from the last thought, there are some people who are wise enough not to be laid back and live in self defeat. They seek out an expert for consultation. This expert might be in their town. He might be online or he may have a program that fit into the need of the seeker. This expert might be a medical doctor or nutritionist. These are the people who are really prepared to change their condition. They are the people that this book is written for.

So, when you read this book, you no longer need to be hopeless about your situation. A solution is closer to you than you can imagine. There are reports that show how a lot of people who were unfit, fat or obese overcame those conditions and started living life with healthier weights. You too can overcome any undesirable fitness and weight conditions and go on to share your own testimony. The information on how to go about this weight reduction journey is plenty both online and offline. The difficulty for you and for most people is picking what will work for them. However, when viewed critically, the problem is more often with the one who is seeking the solution rather than the solution itself. That is something you have to tackle anyhow and this book offers some tips.

So, do you want to remain unfit or you want to be fit. Do you want to remain obese or you want to be slim so you can fit into trendy beautiful clothes. The decision is yours to make and you better be fast about it. Carrying obesity into later years is a serious burden. The burden is social, health and financial. You do not really want that. So, deal with it now. Some form of mental capacity will be needed but it will be fun. Real fun.

4

How Attitude affect your Desire for weight loss and Fitness

I will ask you a question, Have you been sick before? How often have you completed a course of treatment for an ailment after the symptoms have disappeared? Not often. So, why? You got tired, you felt well or some other reasons. This issue of non-compliance is common. It is this same attitude that plays out when we are trying to tackle our weight loss and fitness problems. Having the right attitude can make the difference between success and failure in weight loss matters. The obese person that challenges himself to move in the direction of weight reduction will generally succeed, all things being equal. This cannot be said of the person who exhibits a poor attitude towards his condition.

I also need to warn that there is a danger associated with half measures. When a person refuses to go all out to deal with a situation but chooses to adopt shortcuts, failure and disappointment is not always far. They follow like a shadow. It is the reason why there are treatment failures for some health conditions. Patients will not go through the full course of treatment. As soon as they feel that their health has rebound, even when not restored, they stop treatment. Later, they come down with similar ailments and then, it is seen that the low power medication cannot work. Then they are introduced to a higher power type which may be effective but will carry greater risk of adverse reactions.

When it comes to dealing with obesity, overweight and fitness, the reasons for non-compliance can be a bit different from those adduced for conventional health treatments. In the case of obesity; Surgery, drugs, diets and exercises are sometimes combined to enable proper treatment of the problem and that is where the matter really is. Most people find it hard to follow through on any two combinations of the above treatment method. They may comply with one method but two becomes a chore and to add a third course of treatment just dulls their interests to continue. So, few people go through it. Now, let us look at the common types and see how they impact on overweight and obesity treatment.

Obesity drugs

It is well known by experts that obesity drugs are not met for every obese person. Most are prescribed in the case of extreme obesity or when necessary. The most commonly prescribed drug is phetermine and it is generic and FDA approved to be used for three months. But this may change. It is also common knowledge that obese persons prefer lifestyle changes to drugs. So, this is a real problem for practitioners. Though, it is said that drugs may help an obese person better on the long term, the inculcating of lifestyle changes into treatment along the line cannot be ruled out. The lifestyle change approach take into cognizance the social, psychological and behavioral attitude that result in obesity and being unfit. The tendency to be fat might run in a family but it is the peculiar behavior towards food and life in general that really makes for expression of the obesity.

So, do not tell me that you are fat because it runs in your family. You can step out of that line of being fat and you can start the journey now.

5

Diet or Nutrition

When somebody comes to the point where he feels his weight is now a problem due to extra fat stores in his belly, laps, hips and other parts of the body, he takes a decision to cut down on his calorie intake. Most times, it is after he has been taunted by others or there is a health issue that he comes to this decision. What does he do in other to cut down this intake? He skips meals. He may stop eating certain foods as they are considered not good but then, over-indulge in others. With time, he realizes that he has not lost much. In desperation, he seeks other solutions. He might go to a hospital or go online. He does not know if a dietician or nutritionist exists and some doctors will not tell him anyway. However, he might also come to know a nutritionist. In any case, these sources will provide solution. The solution provided might be substantially different from what he has been doing. But here is the point. **The ability and willingness to follow through on the recommendations given by any of these sources or experts is important.**

The thing about these recommendations is that they mostly come in programs form. It is like you are trying to treat a chronic disease. You know that you need several doses over a period of time. Not only that, you also need to take certain precautions over the period of that

treatment.

In weight loss and fitness, you are dealing with what can be cured provided you are willing to be patient to follow instruction. Why this is vital is because, you do not pile on weight overnight. It is always over a period of time and to deal with it, you also need time. In some cases, you may get results within two to four weeks but the full benefit of results happen over a period of time. Let me repeat. *You did not get to be fat overnight; you cannot get to reasonable fitness overnight.*

It may be that the program should last for six months to one year to get a good result and then to follow a certain diet pattern to prevent excessive weight gain. All programs are not the same. What happens is that only a very small percentage of those who get the program follow it through. Most do not.

That should not be you. When you get such program prescriptions, you must determine in your mind to do what it takes. That is the first thing to do. **Winning first in your mind**. You must determine to follow through on the program no matter how it looks like. You may have got it from a doctor, a nutritionist, or online. Decide to go all the way. It may not be convenient but it may be worth it at the end. What will help you to decide is to have your eyes on the big picture. Who do you want to see in that photograph, that mirror, that video, that public profile? Who do you want to see?

Fat you? Well, some people like themselves fat. To them, it is a sign that they are well fed. But the truth is, we know it is brought about through wrong eating habits mostly.

Beer belly you? It can make you look funny or intimidating. It depends on the area you are.

Big hip and fat lap you? In this case, movement is a chore.

Fat flabby arm you? We know there is no beauty there.

Or a trimmer you. This is what we are about here. And I know you can get there.

You should have that big picture of a fit and trim you. Add slim if you like. It depends on your goals. But you have to set a goal even if you do not usually do so. If possible, get a book or video on goal setting. Follow the lessons and apply them to this situation. You can even have an artistic impression of a fit and trim you. It does not matter. You want to have an inspiration. You need to work the program. That is how you will get result. You need to find a motivation somehow. I tell you; setting a SMART goal and writing it down is a motivation. So, do it. Do not be lazy now, just write it down. Make it simple and achievable. Setting SMART goals is a general rule of goal setting. Let us apply it here.

It means your goals should be:

Specific- you want to achieve a weight reduction of 20lbs.

Measurable- you want to weigh yourself daily and ensure monitoring.

Achievable- you are sure that this can be done and you are motivated enough to have a go at it. Result oriented-you are going to be focused on this goal by eating right and exercising.

Time bound- You hope to achieve this in a month. And I should add that your goals should be short term and long term.

You should have a short term goal first. Let us say you have a goal to lose 25 lbs or 12.5 kg in six months. So, you weigh 250 lb. You want to cut it down by 25 lbs or 12.5kg in six months. That is 10 percent from baseline which is supported by research findings. You will have to break that down into a daily, weekly and monthly goal depending on your available time. After all, you do have a life and there is money to be earned and other matters too. Now, what is your BMI? Is it in the overweight range of 27 to 35 or obesity range

>35. Knowing your BMI will help you to know the calories you should be decreasing both by diet and exercise. Generally, it should be a decrease of 300 kcal to 1000 kcal daily to achieve 10 percent weight decrease in 6 months. Let us say you have a monthly goal overall. You will be aiming to lose about 4.2 pounds or 2 kg per month. This is just an example, mind you. Your goal might even be to lose 40 or 50 lbs in 6 months. The principle is the same. Only some adjustment is required and more sacrifice. It comes down to your attitude.

What then after setting this goal. Faith and Action is required. Persistent action. You must know that to lose weight, you need to consume fewer calories than you burn. To lose say 25 pounds over six months, you will need to cut like 500 to 1000 calories out of your diet. I know, i said it before. It bears repeating. You need to commit to that. You need to weigh yourself daily. Studies show that adults who weigh themselves daily lose weight more than those who do not. And it is best to do it in the morning before any other thing. Weighing yourself is self monitoring. Very important. But what if you are not keen on daily weigh ins. No problem. You can do it twice weekly. Just try and have that goal of losing 25 pounds in front of you and allow yourself to persist in action. That is the only way to win the fight over your excessive weight issues. **Determination, goal setting and persistent action**. If you fail to do this, expect failure. There is no magic to it. Now, note this. Most programs might recommend that you do the weigh in daily. But I did say you can do it twice weekly. Why I said that is just purely a matter of motivation. Some people might not see those little changes that a daily weigh in reads. If they do, it might not look exciting. But when they do it like twice weekly, they might see a bigger change and that might really inspire them to go on. The choice is yours to make anyway.

The program you bought (whether recommended or online) will have a diet segment and maybe an exercise segment. The first thing to do is to look at the **diet** segment. This is because you can begin to deal with it immediately and the diet aspect is the real deal for weight loss or not. Normally, the diet patches will be more than one. Select which one to start with and start working. Ensure you understand what you are doing. If not, ask questions...

Now, experts agree that in-person consultation is better than buying programs. So, it is recommended. Yes, I do recommend it because you get to interface with an expert who can monitor your progress. And that is a big advantage provided you can get that expert. It is like setting a date for a serious test and you prepare as much as you can to pass it. There is that excitement that goes with it and when the day comes, you wonder how you will perform. Now, the fact that you have somebody who can look at what you are doing in an expert way and tell you what you have done right or wrong makes a lot of difference. Frequent contacts with a practitioner during dietary therapy help to promote weight loss and even weight maintenance when you have lost some weight.

But if you are self motivated, and you are sure that you can follow a program and can get someone around you to help in monitoring your progress, then you can also buy a program. Action of any sort is better than nothing.

Having said that, you need to know a bit of information. There are all sorts of diet. Let us look at some. Not in any particular order I should say.

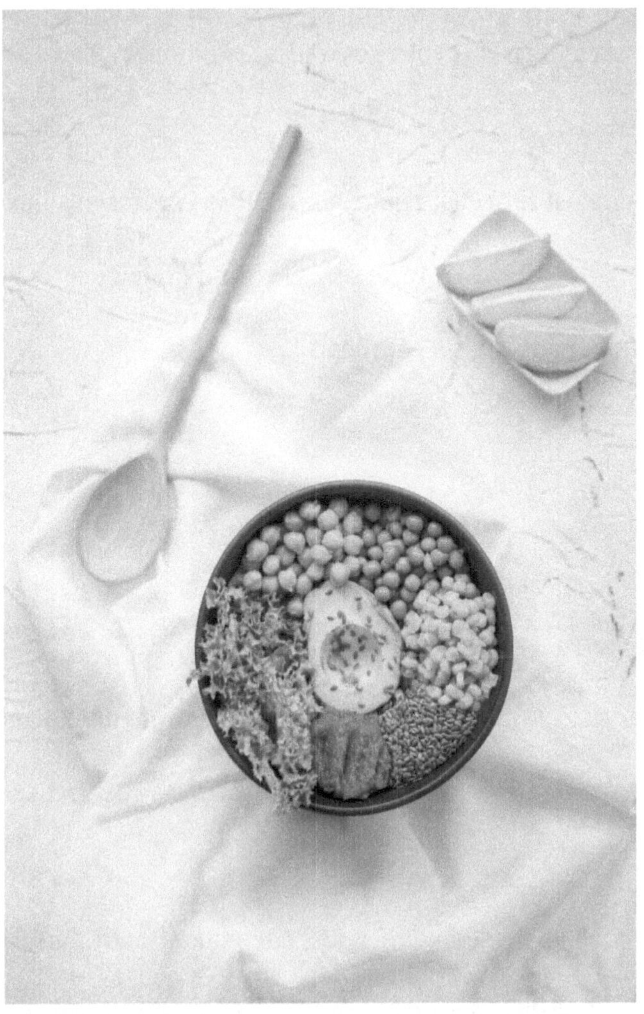

1. Vegetarian diet

There are various types of vegetarian: lacto-vegetarian, fruitarian vegetarian, lacto-ovo vegetarian, living food diet vegetarian, ovo-vegetarian, pesco-vegetarian, and semi-vegetarian.

The majority of vegetarians eat eggs, dairy, and honey. They are lacto-ovo-vegetarians.

Studies over the last few years have shown that vegetarians have a lower body weight, suffer less from diseases, and do have a longer life expectancy than people who eat meat.

2. Ketogenic diet

It is a popular diet. It involves reducing carbohydrate intake and increasing fat intake. It allows the body to burn fat as a fuel, rather than carbohydrates.

Healthy fats, such as those in avocados, coconuts, Brazil nuts, seeds, oily fish, and olive oil are freely added to the diet to maintain an overall emphasis on fat.

The diet causes the breakdown of fat deposits for fuel and creates substances called ketones through a process called ketosis. This diet has risks including ketoacidosis for people with type 1 diabetes however, and may result in diabetic coma and death. Although most studies are 2 years or less, there is some promising research in relation to diabetes management, metabolic health, weight loss, and body composition change.

3. Atkins diet

The Atkins diet, or Atkins nutritional approach, focuses on controlling the levels of insulin in the body through a low-carbohydrate diet.

It is known that if people consume large amounts of refined carbohydrates, their insulin levels rise and fall rapidly. Rising insulin levels trigger the body to store energy from the food that is consumed, making it less likely that the body will use stored fat as a source of energy.

Therefore, people on the Atkins diet avoid carbohydrates but can eat as much protein and fat as they like.

The Atkins Diet comes with certain risks. Individuals considering the Atkins Diet should speak with their doctor.

4. Vegan diet.

A vegan does not eat anything that is animal-based, including eggs, dairy, and honey. I once knew a vegan and I could not understand how somebody could live without eating fish, meat and such other animal based foods. Vegans adopt veganism for health reasons, and also for environmental, ethical, and compassionate reasons.

Vegans believe that if everybody ate plant-based food, the environment would benefit, more food would be produced, and people would generally enjoy better physical and mental health. Of course, animals will not need to be killed or undergo suffering.

5. The Zone diet

The Zone diet aims for a nutritional balance of 40 percent carbohydrates, 30 percent fats, and 30 percent protein in each meal. The focus is also on controlling insulin levels, which may result in more successful weight loss and body weight control than other approaches.

The Zone diet encourages the consumption of high-quality carbohydrates - unrefined carbohydrates, and fats, such as olive oil, avocado, and nuts.

7. South Beach diet

The South Beach diet was started by a cardiologist, Dr. Agatston, and a nutritionist, Marie Almon. It focuses on the control of insulin levels, and the benefits of unrefined slow carbohydrates versus fast carbohydrates. Dr. Agatston devised the South Beach diet during the 1990s because he was disappointed with the low-fat, high-carb diet backed by the American Heart Association. He believed that low-fat regimes were not effective over the long-term.

8. Raw food diet

The raw food diet, involves consuming foods and drinks that are not processed, are completely plant-based, and ideally organic.

Raw foodists believe that at least three-quarters of a person's food intake should consist of uncooked food. A significant number of raw foodists are also vegans and do not eat or drink anything that is animal based.

There are four main types of raw foodists: raw vegetarians, raw vegans, raw omnivores, and raw carnivores.

9. Mediterranean diet

The Mediterranean diet is Southern European, and more specifically focuses on the nutritional habits of the people of Crete, Greece, and southern Italy.

The emphasis is on lots of plant foods, fresh fruits as dessert, beans, nuts, whole grains, seeds, olive oil as the main source of dietary fats. Cheese and yogurts are the main dairy foods. The diet also includes moderate amounts of fish and poultry, up to about four eggs per week, small amounts of red meat, and low to moderate amounts of wine.

Up to one-third of the Mediterranean diet consists of fat, with saturated fats not exceeding 8 percent of calorie intake. This diet is the most extensively studied diet to date, with reliable research supporting its use for improving a person's quality of life and lowering disease risk.

So, there you have it. There are other diet types I did not mention but these are among the popular ones and they can be effective too in dealing with the matter at hand. So, whichever you choose or is recommended for you, you have to be sure you can keep at it for a long time. Whether it is suitable and affordable is a decision you have to make.

6

Exercise

The place of exercise in weight loss, fitness and weight management is well documented. Nothing is really new except a reminder of basic things. Man forgets a lot. Every weight loss and fitness program does include exercise in it. It is not a calculated attempt to gain more on the part of the provider. Exercise is essential to man's existence and is necessary for our overall health. It helps us to maintain our weight and ensure proper body function. A lack of exercise is a recipe for health problems that otherwise should not happen. The point must be made however that exercise in weight loss regimen is more of a balancing of the health than for actual weight loss. There is plenty of science to support that.

In weight loss and fitness regimens, exercises are included to speed up the burning of calories and build muscles. This is achieved because of the balancing effect of proper exercise on the entire body system. This effect results in the proper absorption of nutrients and the transport of waste products out of the cells to appropriate organs of the body for elimination. If you exercise properly, you will observe that you will sweat more; your bowel movement will improve. Your food portions will also change for the better. I am talking of regular exercise here. Same for your food choices. You will just discover that you hate certain wasteful habits like smoking and alcoholism. From experience, when I really go a whole week in performing exercise, I stay clear from any form of stimulant or whatever may have a depressing feeling on me. So, kola nuts, alcohol, plenty coffee or tea is a no for me. I do not even touch cigarettes. I just drink water mostly or some juice. This may not be your case but regular exercise does help one to regulate food and drink intake.

So, exercise is very good for you and that is why it is included in these programs. Exercise effectiveness stems from its effect on adipose tissue by making it perform its fat metabolism and hormonal role. In other words, when you exercise as prescribed for you, you will lose fat and gain muscles. The more you keep at it, the more fats you burn. Do note however that losing fat may not lead to weight loss except you also do something about your diet.

When it comes to exercises, expert advice is needed. In case of mild exercises like brisk walking for a short distance, that advice may not be needed. However, for the types of exercises prescribed in most weight loss programs, you need to seek expert advice. This is necessary if you have other health issues apart from obesity or overweight. And from statistics, anywhere you find obesity; you will find some health issues.

When all these are done, your next action will be to follow the instruction you are given. Just like in the case of the nutrition, you must have **goals, determination and persistent action**. Indeed, these three factors are very important here. You and I know that the last thing on our mind each day is to exercise. That is for professional sports people, not us, we will say or assume. So, we do not really bother until things get out of hand.

When you are obese or overweight, you know that things have gotten out of hand. When your belly begins to sag, you know that things have gotten out of hand. And it is time, to get back in shape. Engaging in exercise does that.

So, what is your exercise goal?

Not every activity that results in sweating is an exercise.

Cooking and sweating,

Eating and sweating,

Gardening and sweating are not the same.

Only the last activity qualifies as an exercise.

Also, results are gotten from a combination of exercises. Engaging in one line of exercise like say, gardening will not give you the desired result whether your goal is weight loss or fitness. You have to combine them as you are instructed. That is the only way you will reap the benefits.

Why is engaging in various exercise necessary. The body is highly intelligent and safety aware. It quickly recognizes a pattern and fit into it. The problem with that is that you feel good but you do not profit from it. Your body like defined pattern. If you want to get the best out of exercises, you must vary them. That way, you confuse the body's memory and you are able to make it release fat stores to fuel the needed calorie demand. When you do this continuously, you keep losing fat stores because your metabolism is balanced in favor of breakdown of fats instead of a buildup of same. So, you can see why every weight loss and management program will always include an exercise component.

Remember, the key is to continue in the process. Even if there is a break, it should not be for too long. It will be good to stick notes to your mirror, reading table, dressing table, even dining table, and to have notes tucked away on whatever you carry often. Say, wallet, handbag. The notes are to remind you of what you must do. The task you must accomplish.

I will advise that these notes should not be the same. Let the notes be on cardboard paper. That way, they wll resist squeezes. And you can easily tuck them into corners and narrow openings. As to what to write; if for instance, a note says *I must exercise for thirty minutes today,* another should say *have you exercised today for thirty minutes* and so on. You should aim to exercise for 200 to 250 minutes per week. Setting a time period is important. It is another way of setting a goal. We all know that goal setting helps. You could not possibly succeed in a situation like this without setting a goal. This is a serious matter not a leisure thing. So, when you get down to doing exercise, use the timing well. You will also remember to do 1-10 counts. You need to have exercise cycles and each cycle will have repeats of activity. It is a good thing to learn to count each rep.

this will force you to be more focused on what you are doing and

after you finished the exercise cycle; you will feel good about

yourself. This feel good factor is a major exercise goal. Anyone who

completes an exercise cycle does feel good about themselves. I am

sure you know how important such a feeling is to anybody.

7

Leverage on Social

Social interaction is important to compliance in weight loss and

fitness exercises. This works even with in-person consultation.

Before I go on here, i want to say that from my experience, the times

I have exercised more was when friends were given me encouragement. There are certain motivations that go with friends encouragements. So, try it. Here is how to go about it. Most programs may not include this aspect but it is important. You have a trusted person or persons you deal with. We all do except, if you are a freaky person. Even if the program is a form of in-person type as I mentioned before, you should still have a third party validation of your effort and progress. This person should be someone who is not afraid to tell you that you are wrong if that opinion is called for.

So, get this person or persons. Show them the program recommended for you. Like I said, it can be offline from a qualified person or online from a weight loss site. I do not care which. Just let the person know what you are about, to get the support you need. State clearly the goals you are trying to achieve. Both the short term goal and the long term. You have to face it. The long term goal is the main thing. You do not want to lose weight or lose fat and then gain everything back and even some more in a short while. You want to maintain a healthy weight and that is only possible with a long term goal. So, avoid programs that promise massive weight loss in a very short time of say, a month. Most are trying to get you in.

You can tell the person that you want to lose 40lbs or 80kg in one year. But you want to go gradually like lose 2-4lbs a month. Do **not** use words like 'I want to lose some so so pounds a day or a week?' You might not be able to meet up and that may frustrate you rather than inspire you. Again, such little changes might not make much impact on you. But if at the end of the month you see that you have lost say 2 lbs out of 4 lbs that you aimed for, you will feel good and might want to try more. In any case, this is my opinion. Generally, success, no matter how small, does inspire us. It cannot be radically different for someone who has a goal of losing weight or slimming down. I know you are still with me.

Again, I want you to remember that it is both the diet and exercise combination that I am talking about here. So, that is also what your friend is helping you to monitor. I know it can be awkward when you have to be answering questions that look silly to you at times.

But this social monitoring system works. It is really what we do. Only that you are applying it to a defined program.

You can even stretch it further by using social media. You can join a similar interest group and explain in simple and plain language what you are about to do. Tell them your weight, height, BMI and other information that will aid them in giving sound advice. Tell where you are now in weight loss treatment and where you want to be. For instance, you could say (------ well I am currently weighing 225 kg, with a BMI of 30. But I am aiming for 170 kg the next one year. Any advice please). You know something like that. Then see those who respond and pick like two that you like for regular communication via private mail. They are the ones you should go into details with.

See, you can use your children to track what you are doing. If you have anyway. Just tell them what you are about and show them what you want them to do.

You should keep a chart of your entire program compliance including how your exercise is going. I know it seem like work but one aspect of weight loss is the ability to engage in activities of various kinds. So, charting your progress is one of such activity. This chart should also include your weight loss progress. You should be reviewing this chart with your helper as often as it is convenient.

A simple chart can have sections like: Date, diet type, weight in, exercise time, others, weight out, remark. The weight in and weight out might not be for a single exercise and prescribed program but for a whole range of time say, one week or a month. But it is good to note the exercise time separately elsewhere and then to add everything up. This chart can be drawn up using paper or cardboard. If you are comfortable using software programs, then use word processor or any of such programs. You do not have to be on the internet to do this. And do be flexible.

See example below.

Table: Weight loss Progress Chart

DATE	DIET TYPE	EXERCISE TYPE	EXERCISE	WEIGHT	REMARK

			TIME	IN/OUT	
9/ **3/17**	KETO	Push up, run for 3km	5:30 am	170/1 69 kg	Slight weight loss.

Another aspect of this social interaction involves telling those close to you to observe you every time to see if there are changes in your bodily make up. It does not mean you have to jettison the first aspect. It is just to have additional independent opinions and also, it helps in situations where you have no one who is willing to go through all the trouble with

Motivation is crucial.

To lose weight and to keep it off, it is vital that you should be motivated to really want to lose weight, and want to improve aspects of your life style. No weight-loss plan will work unless you have a serious desire to lose weight. You may not feel that being overweight or obese is a problem to you. So, you may have little motivation or desire to lose weight. That is fine, so long as you understand the health risks.

For emphasis, let us repeat the health risks of being overweight or obese.

People who are overweight or obese suffer from all forms of health conditions.

All-causes of death (mortality)

High blood pressure (Hypertension)

High LDL cholesterol, low HDL cholesterol, or high levels of triglycerides (Dyslipidemia)

Type 2 diabetes

Coronary heart disease

Stroke

Gallbladder disease

Osteoarthritis (a breakdown of cartilage and bone within a joint)

Sleep apnea and breathing problems

Some cancers (endometrial, breast, colon, kidney, gallbladder, and liver)

Low quality of life

Gynecological abnormalities.

Stress incontinence

Mental illness such as clinical depression, anxiety, and other mental   disorders

Body pain and difficulty with physical functioning

When you consider the above ailments, you know that you need to put in the effort and get the right attitude to effect a change in the quality of your life.

You have to know that certain actions cannot help you to achieve weight loss. The chief culprit here is living a sedentary lifestyle. Overweight and obese people are prone to that.

Lounging in front of the TV while snacking on chips and soda isn't going to reduce your weight. While working up a sweat and changing your eating habits might sound like torture to your predominantly sedentary self, they can help you lose weight. With some effective changes that can still be enjoyable, you'll lead a more active, healthy lifestyle that will make you feel better and look better. Small dietary adjustments can promote weightloss without too much effort on your part; you just have to choose healthy, low-calorie foods, and eat them. Veggies, whole grains, low-fat dairy, lean protein and fruits should be staples in your diet. You can keep excess calories at bay be drinking 2 cups of water or eating a salad or broth-based soup before each meal. This can take the edge off so you're not overindulging in the maincourse. Also, having pre-cut veggies and an low-caldipon hand comes in handy during cravings for unhealthy snack foods.

Conclusion

You do not have to keep that excess weight. You can shed them and become fit and trim. Just as you did not pile up the weight in one day, it is wrong to think you can shed them in one day. It takes time to lose the pounds but you will certainly lose them. Do not doubt that. What you will need is self believe. Whatever system or program you adopt will require work. If you do not work it, it will not work. So, before you spend money further, settle this in your mind.

Remember that losing weight is half the battle, management of your weight is another half. But there is no hard science to it. We all do it without even knowing. We exercise, avoid certain foods, fast, skip some meals, eat small portions, drink lots of water based on how we feel. Overall, our weight is kept from increasing but we usually do not take note. You do take note because; you are coming from a direction of fat to slim. What you should not do is to drop the diet by tricking yourself to it. You have to uphold your routines. To help yourself, be flexible with the diet by altering the diet plan a bit so you can stick with it and be happy. But do not drop it except it feels awful.

Once you achieve your goal, just be reasonable about your lifestyle and be really watchful. You do not want to go back to where you came from.

To your best weight loss success ever.

About The Author

I am just a guy who is schooled in science to degree level . I like to see people live in healthy bodies and in healthy shape. The reason is because majority of people who are out of shape experience low self esteem. I really do like people to esteem themselves highly but not higher than others. You know that is a problem on its own. So, i took to writing this little book with the hope that it may be of help to some people who may care to read it and apply the wisdom it contains. I do hope you will be that person.